TABLE OF CONTENTS

UC/tlk

1

STAYING HEALTHY

SHREWD WAYS TO AVOID A COLD...
WISE WAYS TO TREAT A COLD

Source: **Isadore Rosenfeld, MD,** Rossi Distinguished Professor of Clinical Medicine at Weill Medical College of Cornell University in New York City. He is author of numerous books, including *Dr. Rosenfeld's Guide to Alternative Medicine: What Works, What Doesn't and What's Right for You.* Ballantine Books.

The common cold is caused by any of more than 300 viruses. **YOU CAN PROTECT YOURSELF BY OBSERVING THE FOLLOWING RULES...**

• *Stop stressing yourself out.* Pushing yourself too hard depresses the immune system. When your defenses are down, you are more vulnerable to infection by a cold virus.

Go to sleep at a reasonable hour. A fully rested body is better able to resist infection.

Know your limits—physically and emotionally—and try not to exceed them.

• *Wash your hands* after using staplers, copiers, fax machines and any other common office equipment, especially when any of your coworkers have colds.

Viruses can live on hard surfaces for hours, even days. In fact, you can become infected with a cold virus on an airplane—not from the recirculating air, but from touching the lavatory door. If you can't get to a sink, use an alcohol-based antibacterial gel.

• *Eat wisely.* A healthful diet is especially important to keep your immune system strong. Have the basics—no junk food, lots of fruits and vegetables and plenty of noncaffeinated liquids.

Some doctors recommend 1,000 to 2,000 milligrams (mg) of vitamin C per day to strengthen your defenses against cold viruses. This seems to reduce the severity of cold symptoms.

WHEN YOU FEEL A COLD COMING ON...

• *Take echinacea.* While recent research on hundreds of people found that echinacea was no more effective than a placebo, in my experience it is a very good placebo.

Although the effectiveness of this herb is controversial, many doctors, especially in Europe, believe it can shorten the duration of a cold and lessen the severity of the symptoms.

I prefer the tincture. Take 15 to 20 drops diluted in one-quarter of a glass of water, four times a day. Continue this dosage for about two weeks, if necessary...then stop.

IMPORTANT: *This is not for everyone.* Anyone with immune system disorders, such as lupus or scleroderma, should not take echinacea. Check with your doctor.

TREATING A COLD...

• *Drink hot fluids.* The best liquid for a cold is hot chicken soup. It works more effectively than most other soups—but no one knows exactly why.

Hot tea and steaming lemon-flavored water also keep nasal passages open.

A vaporizer—hot or cold—can provide the same steam-clearing effect in your nasal passages.

• *Take an antihistamine to relieve a stuffy nose.* While antihistamines won't cure a runny nose, their drying effect may make you feel better. They are especially good when there is an allergic component to the cold.

BEWARE: Men with prostate problems may experience difficulty urinating and should avoid antihistamines.

Nasal decongestants that are sold over the counter or nasal sprays can also relieve stuffy nose symptoms.

- *Treat coughs with the right cough medicine.*
  - If you have a cough that is producing phlegm, choose medicine with the ingredient *guaifenesin.* It loosens the mucus that is causing you to cough.
  - If you have a dry, irritating cough that doesn't produce mucus, you may wish to suppress it during the night so you can sleep. Choose a cough medicine with the codeine-like ingredient *dextromethorphan.*
- *Avoid antibiotics—in most cases.* If, however, your cold turns into bronchitis or you have a persistent fever or green sputum, your doctor may then prescribe antibiotics.

■

FOODS THAT HELP HANDLE A COLD

Source: Nutrition for Dummies (For Dummies) by **Carol Ann Rinzler.** She is a New York City–based author of numerous health-related books.

- *Chicken soup* really makes you feel better fast—though researchers do not know why.
- *Sweeteners like honey, molasses and sugar* soothe sore throats.
- *The sour taste of lemon tea and sour-lemon drops* helps saliva flow—and also soothes the throat.
- *Hot peppers, horseradish and onions* make it easier to blow your nose and cough up mucus.

■

GARLIC AND YOUR HEALTH

Source: **John Milner, PhD,** chief, nutritional science research group, division of cancer prevention, National Cancer Institute, Bethesda, MD.

Recent studies conducted in the US, Europe and China suggest that garlic can lower cholesterol levels...fight bacterial and viral infections...prevent cancer...and boost memory.

How strong is the evidence? Could you benefit by adding more garlic to your diet...or by taking garlic pills?

GARLIC VS. CHOLESTEROL...

As proponents of garlic are quick to point out, numerous studies suggest that regular consumption of garlic—one clove a day or the equivalent in supplement form—cuts serum cholesterol by 7% to 15%. Garlic seems to be especially helpful at reducing LDL (bad) cholesterol.

Other studies suggest that garlic has little or no effect on cholesterol levels.

EXAMPLE: A study conducted at the University of Bonn and published in *The Journal of the American Medical Association* showed that cholesterol levels remained unchanged even when garlic oil equivalent to four to five cloves of garlic was consumed on a daily basis for 12 weeks.

What explains the inconsistency of the studies? It may be that only some people respond to garlic. It's also possible that garlic interacts with the other foods in one's diet. In addition, the studies used various garlic preparations. Some used unprocessed garlic. Others used a garlic extract—which may or may not have the same biological activity as whole garlic.

GARLIC VS. CANCER...

Research suggests that garlic can help prevent a variety of malignancies...

• *Stomach cancer.* In a study conducted in China, people who ate garlic regularly had an unusually low rate of this potentially deadly cancer.

• *Colon cancer.* A study of women in Iowa found that the incidence of colon cancer was 50% lower among those who consumed the most garlic.

• *Prostate cancer.* A study conducted in Oxford, England, found that men who consumed garlic two or more times per week were one-third less likely than other men to develop prostate cancer.

If garlic does protect against cancer, the explanation may lie in the sulfur compounds it contains.

Some laboratory studies have demonstrated that these compounds block the synthesis of carcinogens known as *nitrosamines*. In the absence of sulfur, the digestive process leads to the formation of nitrosamines each time nitrates and nitrites are consumed.

Nitrates and nitrites are found in preservatives and in beets, spinach and certain other foods.

Garlic also stimulates the body to synthesize *glutathione.* In addition to deactivating certain carcinogens, this natural antioxidant protects cell membranes against damage caused by renegade molecules known as *free radicals.*

Recent studies suggest that it might be possible to derive cancer chemotherapy drugs from garlic.

HOW TO EAT GARLIC...

There is no *proof* that garlic can reduce cholesterol, lower cancer risk or do anything else to protect your health. But given the evidence in garlic's favor—plus the fact that the only downside to garlic consumption is bad breath—it makes sense to include some in your diet. One to three grams of garlic per day—the equivalent of one clove—should be enough.

If you cook with garlic, be careful to preserve the potentially beneficial sulfur compounds. To do this, peel garlic, chop or crush it and then let it stand for 15 to 30 minutes before cooking. This "waiting period" facilitates chemical reactions that yield the biologically active compounds.

■

ALMONDS CUT CHOLESTEROL

Source: **Gene A. Spiller, PhD,** director of the Sphera Foundation and Health Research and Studies Center, Los Altos, CA.

In a study, 45 people with high cholesterol levels were placed on a diet rich in almonds, olive oil or dairy products.

RESULT: After four weeks, the almond group had LDL (bad) cholesterol levels an average of 16 points lower than the olive oil group...and 33 points lower than the dairy group.

Almonds are rich sources of monounsaturated fats, fiber and the amino acid *arginine.* Each of these contributes to the cholesterol-lowering effect. Even if you are taking cholesterol-lowering medication, consider including almonds in your diet ...along with fruits, vegetables, beans, whole grains and garlic.

■

ESSENTIAL SECRET FOR KICKING ADDICTIONS

Source: **Jamison Starbuck, ND,** a naturopathic physician in family practice and a lecturer at the University of Montana, both in Missoula. She is past president of the American Association of Naturopathic Physicians and a contributing editor to *The Alternative Advisor: The Complete Guide to Natural Therapies and Alternative Treatments.* Time Life.

Addiction to alcohol, tobacco or drugs destroys lives—those of the addicts and those of their friends and family. Short of incarceration, the only way to stop addictive behavior is to decide to stop. Typically, this decision comes after months or years of internal debate. **IF YOU'VE REACHED THIS POINT, I OFFER SEVERAL SUGGESTIONS THAT MIGHT PROVE HELPFUL...**

• *Make a commitment—in writing.* Pick a quit date. Write that date on a piece of paper, along with a written vow to quit, and post it somewhere highly visible. Your vow will be a guidepost, especially in the midst of your journey, when the going gets tough—as it inevitably does.

• *Line up people who will support your decision to quit.* Choose individuals you respect but with whom you have no strong emotional ties. For most people, that means a doctor, clergyman, therapist...and/or maybe an ex-smoker or ex-drinker. Explain your plan, and meet with your support "team" regularly during the withdrawal period.

Spend time with people who encourage your decision to quit—which may mean you'll have to make new friends.

• *Eat according to a schedule.* Eating on a regular basis helps curb your cravings—by keeping blood sugar levels relatively constant. Large swings in blood sugar levels are known to trigger intense cravings—for tobacco and alcohol as well as for food.

I usually advise my patients fighting addictions to eat three meals a day. Each meal should include a small amount of lentils, peas, soybeans or another source of protein. Fresh vegetables and fiber-rich foods like rice, barley, baked potatoes and whole grains are also important during withdrawal. These foods are digested at a slow, steady pace, so they help keep blood sugar levels constant.

• *Consider taking vitamin supplements and herbal remedies.* Vitamin pills will not make quitting easier. But certain vitamins do reduce withdrawal symptoms. I typically recommend 100 milligrams (mg) each of vitamins B-3, B-5 and B-6...400 micrograms (mcg) of vitamin B-12...800 mcg of folic acid...1,000 mg of vitamin C...and 400 international units (IU) of vitamin E—due to possible interactions between vitamin E and various drugs and supplements as well as other safety considerations, be sure to talk to your doctor before starting vitamin E. Supplements should be taken with food on a daily basis.

Herbs, too, can be helpful—especially for people trying to give up smoking. Giving up cigarettes often causes a transient cough and/or lung congestion. A tea made up of mullein, marshmallow root, coltsfoot and peppermint helps keep the lungs clear.

Buy an ounce or two of each herb at a health food store. Mix them in a jar, and use two teaspoons of the herb mix per eight ounces of boiling water. Three cups daily during the first two weeks of quitting should help keep your lungs healthy.

People addicted to alcohol or drugs often benefit from taking milk thistle capsules. This herb helps curb the achy, flu-like symptoms that often strike during withdrawal.

I generally recommend 200 mg to 400 mg of milk thistle to be taken on a daily basis for the first month after the quit date. People with a history of liver disease or who take medication that affects the liver should consult a doctor before using.

■

SUNSHINE REMEDY

Source: **Norman E. Rosenthal, MD,** medical director, Capital Clinical Research Associates (CCRA), Rockville, MD, and clinical professor of psychiatry, Georgetown University, Washington DC. He is author of *Winter Blues.* Guilford Press.

Many people crave sweet and starchy foods during dark winter days because of depressed levels of the brain chemical *serotonin*. The serotonin level can be brought up again by exposure to bright light.

Researchers advise those troubled by cravings for carbohydrates to go outside for 10 minutes to half an hour on sunny winter days if it is not impossibly cold. The most effective time is morning.

■

SUPER FAT-BLOCKER

Source: **Arnold Fox, MD,** an internist and cardiologist in private practice in Beverly Hills, CA. He is coauthor of *The Fat Blocker Diet: The Revolutionary Discovery that Lowers Cholesterol, Reduces Fat, and Controls Weight Naturally.* St. Martin's Press.

In my 40 years of practicing medicine, I've seen every kind of diet aid you can imagine. But when it comes to producing lasting weight loss, I have never seen anything like *chitosan* (KITE-o-san).

This natural food supplement—made from the shells of lobsters—forms a gel in the stomach.

This gel bonds with any fats that are present, forming fatty "clumps" that are indigestible. These clumps pass out of the body in the feces.

Animal studies have shown that chitosan taken before a meal blocks the absorption of up to 50% of consumed fat.

One double-blind study published in Italy found that people who ate a low-fat diet and used chitosan lost an average of 16 pounds...compared with seven pounds for those who followed a low-fat diet without chitosan.

I usually tell my overweight patients to set a target weight, then take 1,000 milligrams (mg) of chitosan 30 minutes before eating lunch and dinner. Once the goal is reached, they can stop taking chitosan.

Taking chitosan does *not* give you permission to eat whatever you want. But it will give you an extra push in the right direction.

There's no evidence that chitosan causes any side effects—but consult your doctor before trying it just to be safe, especially if you're taking any other medications.

CAUTION: Avoid chitosan if you're allergic to shellfish, or are pregnant or breast-feeding. Don't take vitamins A, D or E within four hours of taking chitosan. If you do, the health benefits of these vitamins will be lost.

Chitosan pills are available at most drugstores.

■

FOLATE FINDINGS

Source: **Robert M. Russell, MD,** director of the Jean Mayer USDA Human Nutrition Research Center on Aging at Tufts University, Boston.

Folate—the wonder vitamin—brings dramatic health benefits for women...and men. It prevents birth defects, such as spina bifida, when taken in early pregnancy...and it lowers blood levels of *homocysteine*, an amino acid that in excess increases heart attack risk. Folate, a B-vitamin, also protects against colon and cervical cancers...and treats depression.

BEST SOURCES: Dark green, leafy vegetables...orange juice ...liver...fortified breads and cereals. To be extra safe—especially women contemplating pregnancy—take a multivitamin with 400 micrograms (mcg) of folic acid, which is the synthetic form of folate.

CAUTION: Do not exceed 1,000 mcg a day.

■

VITAMIN WARNING

Source: Study conducted by the staff of the *Tufts University Health & Nutrition Letter,* 10 High St., Suite 706, Boston 02110.

Vitamin supplement pills have very little chance of working if they don't dissolve.

SAFETY: Buy only vitamins with the letters "USP" on the label, which means that they have met US Pharmacopeia standards. In a recent study, five of five USP-labeled vitamin supplements dissolved sufficiently enough to release their contents—but two of five non-USP supplements did not.

■

2

ANTIAGING

ANTIAGING STRATEGIES FOR YOUR BODY, FOR YOUR MIND

Source: **David W. Johnson, PhD,** associate professor of physiology/pharmacology at the University of New England College of Osteopathic Medicine, Biddeford, ME. He is author of *Feel 30 for the Next 50 Years.* Avon Books.

The aging process starts earlier than many people realize. Even if you're only 35 years old and have no symptoms of disease, microscopic damage is already occurring in the cells of your major organs.

But progressive damage to the body can be delayed. A multi-pronged program reduces the risk for heart disease, cancer and other major ailments.

It also slows the rate at which people develop "normal" problems of aging—hearing loss, vision loss, memory problems, etc.

ANTIOXIDANTS...

As you may already know, antioxidants are compounds that deactivate *free radicals,* highly reactive molecules that attack cell membranes, proteins and even our DNA.

Free radicals have been implicated in heart disease, cancer and dementia.

Evidence suggests that free radicals are also responsible for the gradual decline of the immune system, which leaves older people increasingly vulnerable to infection. **THUS FAR, FOUR ANTIOXIDANTS SEEM TO BE ESPECIALLY BENEFICIAL...**

• *Carotenoids.* These fat-soluble antioxidants help protect cell membranes.

To boost carotenoid levels in your body, eat more sweet potatoes and other red and yellow vegetables...and take a supplement containing 50 milligrams (mg) of mixed carotenoids every other day.

• *Vitamin E.* This fat-soluble antioxidant has been shown to protect the heart and the brain...as well as to enhance the immune system.

It's hard to get enough vitamin E from grains and other food sources without also getting too much fat. For this reason, it's best to rely on a supplement.

The usual dosage is 200 international units (IU) per day.

• *Vitamin C.* This water-soluble antioxidant—found primarily in citrus fruits—protects the parts of cells that vitamin E and carotenoids can't reach.

The usual dosage is 500 mg every other day.

• *Selenium.* This mineral, found primarily in seafood and liver, plays a pivotal role in neutralizing free radicals. Yet many Americans are deficient in selenium.

The usual dosage is 200 micrograms (mcg) every other day.

In addition to these antioxidants, it's often a good idea to take supplements of folic acid (1 mg per day)...coenzyme Q-10 (50 mg per day)...and zinc (20 mg per day). Discuss the matter with your doctor.

A STRONG BODY...

Why do people tend to get weaker and more easily fatigued as they grow older? For most of us, it's simply that our muscle mass has gotten smaller.

Aging-related muscle shrinkage is known as *sarcopenia*. Most cases of sarcopenia result not from the passage of time, but from disuse—lack of exercise, in other words.

In addition to maintaining strength and vigor, physical activity lowers the risk for heart disease, diabetes, osteoporosis, depression and certain types of cancer.

Exercise also helps prevent hip fracture, which can be debilitating for older people.

For decades now, doctors have been urging their patients to get regular aerobic exercise. That includes running, fast walking, bicycling, swimming and other activities that raise your pulse for an extended period of time.*

Aerobic exercise is essential, but strength training (weight lifting) is equally important.

Use free weights (dumbbells, barbells, etc.) or exercise machines to build muscle in your arms, legs and torso.

Start with a weight that you can lift eight times in rapid succession. The last two repetitions should cause a burning sensation in your muscles. Pause for three minutes, then do another set. Gradually work your way up to three sets of 15 reps.

A SOUND MIND...

The same antioxidants that help prevent heart disease and cancer—vitamin E in particular—also seem to prevent aging-related changes in the brain. Check with your doctor for the dosages that are right for you.

There's no indication that antioxidants improve thinking ability. But research on a family of cognition-enhancing compounds known as *nootropics* (Greek for "mind turning") has shown that these compounds can improve memory in certain individuals.

Two nootropics—each sold over-the-counter—seem especially beneficial...

• **Ginkgo biloba.** This herbal extract has been shown to improve memory and shorten reaction times in people with Alzheimer's disease. Evidence is not as strong, however, in healthy individuals.

TYPICAL DOSAGE: 100 mg twice a day.

*Your goal in doing aerobic exercise should be to raise your heart rate to 50% to 80% of its maximum for at least 20 minutes a day, at least three days a week. To calculate your maximum heart rate, subtract your age in years from 220.

• *Phosphatidylserine.* This compound, derived from plants, helps stabilize cell membranes in the brain and facilitates communication between brain cells (neurons).

Researchers have noted improvements in attention, memory and concentration in individuals who take phosphatidylserine on a daily basis.

TYPICAL DOSAGE: 100 mg twice a day.

"Use it or lose it" applies to the brain as well as to the muscles. Solving complex problems, memorizing things and otherwise giving your brain a workout seem to stimulate neurons to form new connections.

This process helps compensate for the neurons that die or become dysfunctional each day.

If your daily life involves little short-term memory skills, add "memory games" to your routine.

EXAMPLE: After watching the nightly news on television, see how many of the stories you can recall. Have a family member keep track of how you do.

HOW ABOUT HORMONES?...

As estrogen and testosterone levels dwindle, so does the sex drive.

Falling levels of *human growth hormone* (hGH) cause muscle wasting.

Declines in the hormone *DHEA* have been linked to declining energy levels, memory loss and reduced immunity.

Hormone replacement therapy can restore vitality for some people—particularly older people whose levels have dropped significantly. But it requires close medical supervision.

That's true for hGH, DHEA, testosterone and estrogen. Used unwisely, hormone replacement therapy can promote the growth of prostate cancer and breast cancer.

ANTIAGING HELP...

If you'd like to find a physician who can tailor an aggressive antiaging program specifically for you, contact the American Academy of Anti-Aging Medicine at 773-528-4333, *www.world health.net.*

■

MEMORY-BOOSTING MARVEL

Source: **Dharma Singh Khalsa, MD**, president and medical director of the Alzheimer's Prevention Foundation, Tucson. He is author of *Brain Longevity: The Breakthrough Medical Program that Improves Your Mind and Memory.* Warner Books.

If you've begun to experience problems with your memory, ask your doctor about taking *phosphatidylserine.*

This compound occurs naturally in the outer membranes of brain cells...and in certain plants as well.

In recent studies sponsored by the National Institutes of Health, phosphatidylserine improved memory and concentration in people suffering from age-related memory loss and even early-stage Alzheimer's disease.

Phosphatidylserine seems to work just as well as *tacrine* (Cognex) and *donepezil* (Aricept), the only approved prescription medications for Alzheimer's.

Tacrine can cause liver damage. Phosphatidylserine is free of harmful side effects.

For otherwise healthy individuals who simply want to hone their mental skills, I often recommend one 100-milligram (mg) capsule of phosphatidylserine per day.

For mild to severe memory impairment, two or three capsules a day often work better. There is no additional benefit to taking more than 300 mg a day.

Phosphatidylserine can also be taken in conjunction with *ginkgo biloba.* It's usually best to take 40 mg of ginkgo for every 100 mg of phosphatidylserine.

Phosphatidylserine and ginkgo biloba are sold in health food stores.

CAUTION: Consult your doctor before taking ginkgo if you're taking aspirin, *warfarin* (Coumadin) or another blood-thinning drug. Pregnant women should avoid both phosphatidylserine and ginkgo.

■

THE EYES HAVE IT

Source: **Johanna M. Seddon, MD,** director, epidemiology unit, Massachusetts Eye and Ear Infirmary, Harvard Medical School, Boston, quoted in *Third Age News Service,* distributed by Universal Press Syndicate, 4520 Main St., Kansas City, MO 64111.

The foods you eat may play a role in preserving your eyes as you age. *Age-related macular degeneration* (AMD) is the leading cause of vision loss among people over 65, and begins to develop in people as young as 40. It is a gradually developing, painless condition that results in the loss of the ability to see detail. Research suggests that diet might reduce the risk of developing AMD.

RECOMMENDED: A diet with a variety of fruits and vegetables, including dark green leafy vegetables.

■

ANEMIA FIGHTER

Source: **Robert M. Russell, MD,** director of the Jean Mayer USDA Human Nutrition Research Center on Aging at Tufts University, Boston.

People over age 50 should take supplements containing vitamin B-12. A large percentage of people over 50 are unable to extract the necessary amount of this vitamin from food because they do not produce enough stomach acid.

The National Academy of Sciences recommends taking vitamin supplements and/or consuming fortified foods, which are more easily absorbed.

Two daily servings of some fortified breakfast cereals would supply the correct amount of B-12. The recommended daily allowance for people over 50 is 2.4 micrograms (mcg)—contained in multivitamin supplements for older people. A vitamin B-12 deficiency can lead to anemia and nerve damage.

■

3

FIGHTING DISEASE

THE WHOLE TRUTH ABOUT DIETARY FIBER... AND ITS ROLE IN PREVENTING CANCER, HEART DISEASE AND DIABETES

Source: **David J.A. Jenkins, MD, PhD, DSc,** Canada research chair in nutrition and metabolism, department of nutritional sciences, University of Toronto.

For decades, doctors have been assuring their patients that a high-fiber diet could reduce the risk for colon cancer.

Then a study published in an issue of *The New England Journal of Medicine* indicated that fiber appeared to make no difference at all.

Researchers followed 89,000 women for 16 years. They found that those who consumed moderate amounts of fiber developed colon cancer at the same rate as those who ate a diet low in fiber.

Many people were stunned by the study. Consumers began wondering whether all those years of eating bran cereal had been worth the trouble.

KINDS OF FIBER...

Dietary fiber refers to any of the indigestible portions of plant foods we eat. Although we talk about fiber as a single entity, there are actually many kinds of fiber. **THE DIFFERENT TYPES OF FIBER CAN BE GROUPED INTO TWO BROAD CLASSES...**

• *Soluble fiber* dissolves in water, forming a gel. It is found in high amounts in fruits, oats and beans.

• *Insoluble fiber* does not dissolve in water. Instead, it absorbs water to become bulky, which increases the weight of feces and the speed at which waste passes through the intestines and out of the body. Insoluble fiber is found in vegetables, wheat bran and whole grains.

Typically, of all the fiber eaten, two-thirds is insoluble and one-third is soluble.

WHAT FIBER CAN DO...

The same study that found that fiber did not protect against colon cancer showed resoundingly that eating a high-fiber diet helped prevent heart disease and diabetes.

How fiber in the diet helps prevent heart disease is poorly understood. It may alter clotting factors in blood, reducing the risk of *thrombosis*—blockage in an artery that can cause a heart attack.

Fiber may also lower cholesterol levels by reducing the rate at which fatty deposits form within arteries.

Normally, we excrete small amounts of cholesterol in the feces. Soluble fiber binds more cholesterol as bile acids and carries it out of the body.

High-fiber foods protect against diabetes, a major cause of health problems in Western countries. Exactly how fiber helps prevent diabetes remains unknown.

Fiber also guards against....

• *Diverticular disease.* Fiber is the standard treatment for the prevention of *diverticula*. Those are small sacs that balloon out from the colon wall as a result of pressure exerted by feces and intestinal gas.

• *Constipation and hemorrhoids.* Fiber makes stools softer and more bulky. That allows them to pass easily out of the body without the need for straining.

• *Obesity.* High-fiber foods tend to be lower in fat and calories than low-fiber foods. And because fiber adds indigestible bulk, it makes you feel fuller longer.

WHAT ABOUT COLON CANCER?...

Despite *The New England Journal of Medicine* study, it's premature to write off fiber as a means of reducing colon cancer risk.

The average American consumes about 15 grams (g) of fiber a day. For the past 10 years, researchers have been saying that we should be getting at least twice as much fiber. A truly high-fiber diet may contain 40 to 60 g of fiber a day.

In *The New England Journal* study, women who ate the most fiber got only about 25 g a day. Obviously, that's less than the recommended level of fiber intake—and far short of a real high-fiber diet.

BOTTOM LINE: This study did not really investigate the effects of a high-fiber diet.

DIETARY RECOMMENDATIONS...

For most people, it's not especially difficult to obtain 30 to 40 g of fiber per day from food sources. **HERE'S A WORKABLE STRATEGY...**

• *Start each day with a high-fiber breakfast cereal,* such as All-Bran or Fiber One. Add these to your usual cereal until you get used to the taste and texture, then make the transition, gradually, to the high-fiber cereal only.

• *Substitute whole wheat products for white flour products—* bread, pasta, bagels, crackers, etc.

• *Eat at least five servings of fruits and vegetables a day.* Seven servings is better, and 10 will easily put you in the high-fiber range.

• *Eat at least one serving of peas or beans every day.*

Fiber supplements should not be used instead of a proper diet. But the supplements can be beneficial when used in addition to such a diet.

One good fiber supplement is *psyllium*, which is found in Metamucil and other products. High in soluble fiber, psyllium has been found to lower serum cholesterol...flatten blood glucose levels after meals...and keep insulin levels from rising too high. You can dissolve Metamucil in water and drink it...or sprinkle it on breakfast cereal or other foods.

■

A GOOD WRINKLE ON RAISINS

Source: **Gene A. Spiller, PhD,** director of the Sphera Foundation and Health Research and Studies Center, Los Altos, CA.

Raisins could help to prevent colon cancer. They contain a compound that helps the colon get rid of waste more efficiently...and this keeps the colon healthy. The compound—*tartaric acid*—is found mainly in raisins and grapes. Raisins are also high in potassium and protective antioxidants.

■

SELENIUM WARNING

Source: The late **Victor Herbert, MD,** former professor of medicine, Mount Sinai School of Medicine, New York City, and former chief, Hematology and Nutrition Research Laboratory, Veterans Affairs Medical Center, Bronx, NY.

Taking selenium to protect against prostate cancer can be dangerous. While a Harvard study found that daily selenium supplements may result in a reduced risk of advanced prostate cancer, the study failed to look at the incidence of other kinds of cancer. It also did not look at overall death and illness rates. So the study is a mere question mark.

ALSO: There is little evidence that Americans are deficient in selenium. Excessive supplemental doses can lead to nausea, abdominal pain, diarrhea, fatigue and even death.

■

NATURAL CANCER FIGHTER

Source: **Zbigniew Walaszek, PhD,** a scientist at AMC Cancer Research Center, Denver, an independent, not-for-profit research institution focused solely on cancer prevention and control.

The nutrient *glucarate* is a powerful, natural cancer fighter. It can detoxify cancer-causing agents from the environment, such as the carcinogens in barbecued meat. In recent studies, it dramatically reduced the incidence of breast, colon, prostate, lung and other cancers—in some cases by more than half.

RICH SOURCES: Apples...bean sprouts...broccoli...brussels sprouts...cabbage...cauliflower...grapefruit.

BEST: A daily supplement of 1,000 to 2,000 milligrams (mg). Capsules are available at health food stores and pharmacies—but talk with your doctor first. Glucarate has no known side effects, and your body will excrete any excess.

■

HEART HELPER

Source: **Eric B. Rimm, ScD,** associate professor of epidemiology and nutrition at Harvard School of Public Health, Boston. His 14-year study of more than 80,000 women was published in *The Journal of the American Medical Association,* 515 N. State St., Chicago 60610.

Folic acid isn't the only B-vitamin that benefits the heart. Vitamin B-6 does, too.

RECENT FINDING: Women who consumed the most folic acid had a 31% lower risk for heart attack than those who consumed the least. The women who consumed the most B-6 cut their heart attack risk by 33%. Those who consumed high levels of both vitamins reduced overall risk by 45%. Good sources of B-6 include wheat germ, yellowfin tuna and potatoes.

■

PEANUTS VS. HEART DISEASE

Source: **Penny Kris-Etherton, PhD, RD,** distinguished professor of nutrition at Pennsylvania State University, University Park. Her study comparing five types of diets was presented at Experimental Biology meetings in San Francisco.

Peanuts work as well as olive oil to protect against heart disease.

People with mildly elevated cholesterol whose cholesterol-lowering diets included peanuts and peanut butter, and others who used peanut oil, achieved an 11% drop in total cholesterol and a 14% to 15% drop in LDL or "bad" cholesterol.

Those were the same results that were achieved by people using an equal amount of olive oil in their diets. The results are better than those from classic low-fat diets, which can also decrease HDL or "good" cholesterol.

■

EAT AWAY ARTHRITIS

Source: **Lauri M. Aesoph, ND,** a naturopathic physician in Sioux Falls, SD. She is author of *How to Eat Away Arthritis.* Prentice Hall.

Cayenne, ginger and turmeric can bring marked relief from arthritis pain.

These spices work by blocking the release of *substance P,* a brain chemical that transmits pain signals and activates inflammation in the joints.

IMPORTANT: If you decide to begin "spice therapy," let your doctor know—so he/she can adjust your arthritis medication.

• *Cayenne.* Cayenne can be eaten as a spice...or applied in cream form to painful joints. In one study, up to 80% of arthritis patients were helped by an over-the-counter cream containing cayenne pepper extract (capsaicin).

Capsaicin cream is sold in drugstores under the brand names Capzasin-P, Pain Free, Recapsin and Zostrix.

CAUTION: Applying the cream to broken skin can cause pain. Also—don't eat cayenne if you have an ulcer.

• *Ginger.* In a study, ginger eased pain and swelling in 75% of arthritis patients. You can add fresh gingerroot to your cooking. Or you can take one to three gingerroot capsules a day.

CAUTION: Consuming more than 3 grams (g) of ginger at a time can cause stomach upset.

• *Turmeric.* This spice contains *curcumin,* a compound that reduces swelling. In one study, arthritis patients took either 1,200 milligrams (mg) of curcumin or 300 mg of the arthritis drug *phenylbutazone.* Both groups showed comparable improvement in symptoms, but the drug caused side effects.

Cook with turmeric...or take two curcumin capsules three times daily.

CAUTION: Limit daily turmeric consumption to one meal... or six capsules.

■

GREASING THE WHEELS

Source: **Parveen Yaqoob, DPhil,** department of food science and technology, University of Reading, UK.

Rheumatoid arthritis sufferers often find relief by replacing the fats in their diet with olive oil or other monounsaturated oils.

When researchers put 30 men on a diet high in olive oil, they found that after two months their immune systems had a lower level than normal of a molecule that is involved in the inflammation and pain of arthritic joints.

IMPORTANT: The beneficial effect does not come from increasing the amount of olive oil in the diet, but from using it in place of other oils. Other monounsaturated fats like *canola* oil (also called *rapeseed* oil) may produce similar results.

■

OSTEOPOROSIS BREAKTHROUGHS— NEW TREATMENTS CAN PREVENT AND EVEN REVERSE BONE LOSS

Source: **Harris McIlwain, MD,** who specializes in the prevention and treatment of osteoporosis. He is coauthor of *The Osteoporosis Cure: Reverse the Crippling Effects with New Treatments.* Avon.

Age-related thinning of the bones—osteoporosis—is a major health problem. It vastly increases the risk of broken hips, ribs, pelvis and other weakened bones.

It is osteoporosis that leads to the stooped posture associated with advanced age.

CAUSE: An accumulation of small fractures in the vertebrae.

NEW HOPE FOR AGING BONES...

A program of dietary supplements, exercise and bone-restoring medication makes it possible to minimize bone-density loss due to aging. It's even possible to increase your bone density. Best of all, these treatments are effective at any age and it's never too late to start.

CHECKING BONE DENSITY...

In the past, doctors waited until an actual bone fracture occurred in an elderly person before worrying about osteoporosis. But they now realize that the best approach is to address the problem of bone loss much earlier in life, by starting to check the bone density of people at risk for bone loss in middle age.

By detecting and treating bone loss when it first begins, in people's 40s and 50s, we can hopefully prevent age-related bone fractures from happening at all.

The first crucial step is to take a bone density test. This easy, inexpensive procedure can often be done right in your doctor's office (if not, you'll be referred to a lab).

The simplest test, used as a prescreen, measures the density of the wrist and/or heel using a technique called DXA, or *dual-energy X-ray absorptiometry.* If bone loss is indicated, the next step is to do a more definitive DXA test of your hip and lumbar spine.

WHO SHOULD GET A BONE DENSITY TEST?...

Despite the increasing availability of bone density tests, only about 10% of Americans with osteoporosis ever have their bone density evaluated and treated.

You should have a bone density test done if *two or more* of the following risk factors are present...

• *You've had a bone fracture after age 40.*

• *You're a postmenopausal Caucasian woman who isn't taking estrogen.*

• *You smoke cigarettes.*

• *You are over 50 years of age.*

• *You have a relative, such as a parent or grandparent, who had osteoporosis.*

• *You are taking a bone-thinning medication* (cortisone-type drugs or antacids containing aluminum).

PREVENTION AND TREATMENT OF OSTEOPOROSIS...

The key is to retain as much of your "peak bone mass" as possible, through a bone-building calcium-rich diet, exercise and—if necessary—medication. **PREVENTION STRATEGIES...**

• *Eat a diet high in calcium and vitamin D.* A sufficient daily calcium intake is essential for maintaining bone density. Adult women should get at least 1,200 milligrams (mg) of calcium each day (men can get by with slightly less), but the daily requirement jumps back up to 1,500 mg when women reach menopause.

HEALTHY CALCIUM SOURCES: Skim or low-fat milk (300 mg of calcium per one eight-ounce glass), nonfat yogurt, low-fat cheese, soy products, salmon (with bones), sardines, the leafy green vegetables such as broccoli and kale, baked beans and calcium-enriched juices and breads.

• *Take a calcium supplement.* Since postmenopausal American women consume just 800 mg of calcium a day on average—700 mg below their daily requirement—calcium supplements are necessary to ensure strong bones.

The problem with antacids containing calcium carbonate or calcium phosphate, which many women use as calcium supplements, is that only two-fifths of this calcium is absorbed. (You'll get only 200 mg of calcium from a 500 mg antacid tablet.)

Calcium citrate tablets are more effective. Calcium citrate is 60% more "bioavailable" than calcium carbonate or phosphate.

CAUTION: Space out your calcium tablets during the day (high doses taken at one time aren't absorbed as well as smaller doses taken several hours apart). Always take them with meals or a snack (but not with whole-grain cereal or other high-fiber foods, since fiber blocks calcium absorption).

ALSO: Never take calcium at the same time as an iron supplement since the two minerals will bind together, limiting the absorption of both.

• *Be sure you get enough vitamin D.* You need a certain amount of vitamin D a day to facilitate calcium absorption. Most people get this from sunlight (15 minutes a day is enough), but as people age, the skin is less efficient at absorbing sunlight—and less efficient at converting it to vitamin D.

For this reason, doctors suggest people over age 65 take an 800 international unit (IU) daily supplement of vitamin D. Some experts recommend starting even earlier, at age 50.

• *Do weight-bearing exercise.* While calcium helps build bone, several days a week of weight-bearing exercise is also needed to stimulate the bone-building cells to do their work. (This is why even young astronauts start to lose bone mass in space.)

Exercise could include walking, biking, low-impact aerobics, tennis, stair-climbing or rowing. Exercises to strengthen the back and legs are also frequently recommended, since muscle strength has been linked to stronger bones.

• *Avoid cigarettes and moderate your alcohol intake.* For reasons not yet known, the chemicals in cigarette smoke hasten bone loss, making smokers two times more vulnerable to osteoporosis than the rest of the population.

Alcohol's effects are more mixed. Light consumption (one drink a day) appears to boost bone density slightly—but more than three drinks a day will lower your bone density and contribute to osteoporosis.

• *Take estrogen or another bone-building medication after menopause.* For postmenopausal women, hormone replacement therapy (HRT) is the single most effective way to prevent—or at least greatly delay—osteoporosis. However, because of safety concerns—an increased risk of heart disease, stroke and breast cancer—unless your risk for osteoporosis is very high, most doctors will not recommend HRT. At menopause, it's a good idea to discuss with your doctor the benefits and risks of HRT.

Alternative bone-building medications are now available, including Fosamax (effective in 86% of cases) and Evista.

■

VITAMIN E VS. ALZHEIMER'S

Source: **Costas Lyketsos, MD,** professor of psychiatry and behavioral sciences at Johns Hopkins Bloomberg School of Public Health, Baltimore.

Vitamin E may play a role in delaying the progression of Alzheimer's disease. *Dose for healthy people:* 400 international units (IU) daily. *Dose for those with Alzheimer's:* 1,000 to 2,000 IU daily.

CAUTION: Due to possible interactions between vitamin E and various drugs and supplements as well as other safety considerations, be sure to check with your doctor, before starting a vitamin E regimen.

NOTE: A study found that Alzheimer's patients have low blood levels of vitamin B-12 and folate. But it is unclear if these deficiencies are a cause or a consequence, so there is no current reason to take supplements of these nutrients.

■

DIABETIC HEALTH

Source: **Emmanuel Opara, PhD,** associate research professor of experimental surgery and cell biology at Duke University Medical Center, Durham, NC.

Antioxidant vitamins can keep diabetics healthier. A study of 50 Type-2 (non-insulin-dependent) diabetics found that those who showed indications of developing blindness, kidney failure and early death had significantly lower levels of antioxidants in their blood than those who had no such indications. Researchers recommend that diabetics keep up their antioxidant level with a daily dose of vitamin C (500 milligrams [mg]) and vitamin E (800 mg), two powerful antioxidant vitamins. Check with your doctor for the dosages that are right for you.

■

4

RELAXATION

NATURAL REMEDIES TO SOOTHE STRESS... EASE ANXIETY

Source: **Andrew L. Rubman, ND,** associate professor of clinical medicine at I.W. Lane College of Integrative Medicine, Winter Park, FL. He is also medical director of the Southbury Clinic for Traditional Medicines, Southbury, CT.

As we age, we become even more vulnerable to the effects of emotional and physical stress.

Excessive stress can lead to chemical imbalances in the brain and overreactions in its alarm center. This produces a hyper-aroused or anxious state.

If you're suffering from frequent bouts of anxiety, your body and mind are signaling that they need more downtime to restore balance.

INITIAL STEPS...

• *Take frequent time-outs.* Throughout the day, we're confronted with stressful situations. It is critical not to let this stress build up.

For every 50 minutes you work, take a 10-minute break to reduce your stress level. This can actually make you more productive than working straight through. During at least one of these breaks, do deep breathing.

HELPFUL: Inhale slowly, allowing the air to push out your abdomen. Exhale slowly, allowing the stomach protrusion to return to normal. For maximum oxygenation and benefit, each exhalation should last twice as long as each inhalation.

• *Reduce caffeine intake.* In small, irregular doses, caffeine can be medicinal. It increases bile flow, which stimulates the gall bladder and reduces cholesterol. But in regular doses, it can hinder a number of body systems that are responsible for responding to stress.

IMPORTANT: Limit intake to one to two caffeinated drinks a week.

• *Exercise regularly.* Physical activity is necessary to remove waste products, particularly lactic and uric acids, from the muscles and nervous system.

In excess, these acids help make you feel edgy. Mild to moderate activity can both prevent and reduce anxiety for up to two hours.

HELPFUL: Engage in at least 10 to 15 minutes of activity in the morning and afternoon. A brisk walk combined with deep breathing is ideal.

• *Work hard to sleep well.* Irregular sleep patterns and poor-quality sleep confuse your body. Your body becomes less able to respond appropriately to stress, and you are more vulnerable to anxious feelings.

HELPFUL: Keep a regular bedtime, even on weekends. Take a hot bath or a brisk walk three hours before bedtime to prime your body for sleep. Avoid naps. Avoid eating heavy meals or consuming alcohol or caffeine in the evening.

NATURAL SUPPLEMENTS...

A number of nonprescription supplements have now been shown to reduce mild to moderate anxiety. Before you try any vitamin, mineral or herb treatment to modulate symptoms, check with your doctor. Be sure you don't have any medical conditions—including pregnancy and nursing. Ask your doctor if you are taking any drugs that could make a natural remedy dangerous. Experiment with one remedy at a time.

REASON: If you start taking several supplements and develop side effects, you won't know which one is responsible.

You can purchase quality herbs through a licensed naturopathic physician or at a health food store.

Take the herbs listed below daily for three months and then take a two-week break. This strategy will minimize the potential for adverse effects and the risk of becoming psychologically dependent on them.

Natural treatments to ease anxiety (they can be combined but only with the guidance of a licensed naturopathic physician)...

• *B vitamins.* The B vitamins—particularly B-6 and B-12—help regulate the body's response to stress and maintain a healthy nervous system.

WHAT I RECOMMEND TO MY PATIENTS: Twice a day, take a vitamin B complex formula that contains at least 25 milligrams (mg) of B-6...and also contains 1 mg of B-12.

Because these vitamins work best in combination with other nutrients, also take a multivitamin-mineral supplement twice a day.

BEST: Look for B-12 in the form of *hydroxocobalamin* or *methylcobalamin.* They are better absorbed than the more commonly available *cyanocobalamin.*

• *St. John's wort.* This herb works as an antidepressant. It also relieves chronic anxiety. You must take it for several weeks before you feel its effects.

Research shows it lowers anxiety levels as well as Valium without fogging thinking. It decreases the uptake (rate of removal) of serotonin in the brain, thereby increasing serotonin levels, which induces calm feelings. It is not addictive and has few side effects.

WHAT I RECOMMEND TO MY PATIENTS: Take 300 mg of the fresh freeze-dried extract as needed. Avoid so-called "standardized" products. The active ingredients often are not standardized.

WARNINGS: Don't take St. John's wort if you're on an antidepressant, particularly Nardil or Parnate. And—because St. John's wort may make you more sensitive to the sun, always wear sunscreen when you are outdoors.

• *Valerian.* This is a natural sedative—the most popular one used in Europe. It contains ingredients similar to those found in Valium. It is useful for relieving anxiety because it helps you sleep. It isn't addictive, nor does it make you feel groggy the next morning as sleeping pills can.

WHAT I RECOMMEND TO MY PATIENTS: One 150-mg capsule twice a day. Even this low dose can make you drowsy. If you would prefer to take it just for sleep, take one 300-mg capsule one hour before bedtime. It may take several weeks before you notice an improvement in sleep.

WARNING: Don't use valerian if you're taking sedatives, such as phenobarbital or benzodiazepines.

■

FOODS THAT RELAX YOU

Source: **Annemarie Colbin,** certified health education specialist and founder of the Natural Gourmet Institute for Food and Health, New York City. She is author of the chapter "Food for Relaxation" in *The Big Book of Relaxation* (The Relaxation Company) and author of *Food and Our Bones* (Plume).

You probably know that foods rich in carbohydrates and fiber—and *free* of hydrogenated fat (the fat in fried foods, margarine, shortening)—help you stay healthy. But—did you know the same foods also help your mind and body relax?

Steamed vegetables, fruits, whole wheat bread, brown rice, polenta or oatmeal help you relax by providing your body with a source of energy that is steadily metabolized and continuously absorbed—and by stimulating the relaxing brain chemical *serotonin*.

When these foods are consumed with some protein—fish or chicken—they leave you feeling calm and focused.

FOOD MYTHS...

Refined sugar and alcohol *seem* to have a relaxing effect on the body. In fact, they often make you sleepy. But don't be fooled.

After the initial ease of tension, the effects of alcohol wear off, leaving many people tense and angry.

The same is true for sugar. After an initial sugar "rush"—the surge that leaves you feeling temporarily alert and clear-headed—many people feel exhausted.

They typically crave more sugar to get them going again, and a cycle of highs and lows becomes a way of life.

RELAXING FOODS...

To keep your energy in balance and feel tension-free, eat a variety of the following healthful foods...

• *Breakfast.* Start your day with a small piece of fish with dark rye bread...an organic egg on whole-grain toast...or oatmeal cooked with raisins and cinnamon and topped with toasted sunflower and pumpkin seeds.

The protein/carbohydrate combination will leave you feeling relaxed and focused—unlike a high-fat, high-sugar breakfast (a donut or muffin), which may create a need for caffeine and more sugar as the morning wears on.

In general, I don't recommend eating dairy products. Among other things, they tend to make some people feel heavy and congested.

• *Lunching out.* Have a sandwich on whole-wheat bread or pita, an English muffin or rye toast.

GREAT FILLERS: Thinly sliced natural meats like turkey, chicken breast or roast beef...a dab of mustard or a bit of mayonnaise...and vegetables like lettuce, tomato, onion, grated carrots or sprouts.

Another good lunch option is soup—anything with dried beans or peas, such as split pea, lentil, Yankee bean or black bean. Also good are hearty vegetable soups and chicken soup, served with bread and salad.

If your goal is to be alert and energetic, have more protein and fewer carbohydrates for lunch.

GOOD CHOICE: Broiled fish or grilled chicken and a side salad. Avoid dessert.

POOR CHOICE: Pasta and green salad—it's likely to leave you feeling relaxed and ready for a siesta, not raring to go.

• *Lunch at home.* Mash avocado with a little salsa and eat it on whole-wheat pita bread. Mash canned salmon or sardines with some lemon juice, chopped onion and celery and spread on rye crackers.

ONE POTATO: A great low-fat, relaxing side dish or snack is a baked yam or sweet potato. To keep yams on hand, bake six at a time in a 400-degree oven for one hour—but don't wrap or puncture the skin. Store them in the refrigerator and serve cold, sliced and steamed, grilled or pan-fried.

• *Dinner out.* For a good night's sleep, choose pastas (skip the heavy Alfredo sauce), polenta, rice dishes, cooked vegetables, salads, curries, baked or broiled fresh fish...and other dishes that are low in protein and high in complex carbohydrates.

DESSERT: Something fruit-based, like sorbet. Avoid chocolate, which contains caffeine and sugar.

• *Dinner at home.* A high-fiber vegetarian dinner cooked at home will relax you and give you the nutrients you need.

GOOD CHOICES: Brown rice, barley, polenta, kasha, bean soups, green vegetables such as broccoli, baked yams or squash, salad.

DESSERT: Something sweetened with fruit juice, barley malt or maple syrup (which has the added benefit of being high in calcium).

FOODS TO AVOID...

Some foods and drinks stimulate the nervous system and cause tension and insomnia—whether they're consumed in the morning or at night. TO STAY RELAXED, AVOID...

• *Caffeine.* Caffeine-containing foods and beverages include sodas, chocolate, teas—even green tea—and some over-the-counter and prescription medications.

• *Alcohol.* It's OK to have a glass of wine occasionally with dinner, but alcohol every day can interfere with sleep and cause mood swings.

• *Sugar.* When you crave something sweet, try a dessert sweetened with fruit juice, grain malt or maple syrup. Chamomile tea with honey is relaxing. ANOTHER OF MY FAVORITE SWEETS IS BANANAS VERMONT...

4 bananas, ripe but firm
1 tbsp. unsalted butter
1 tbsp. maple syrup
2 tbsp. water

Peel bananas, cut once in half across, then cut each piece in half again lengthwise. Melt the butter and put into a 9" x 14" baking pan. Arrange the bananas in it, turning once to get a little butter on the other side. Mix water and maple syrup and drizzle over the bananas. Broil five minutes, or until bananas soften. Four pieces per person. Serves four.

■

CONTROLLING ANXIETY WITHOUT ANTIANXIETY DRUGS

Source: **Harold H. Bloomfield, MD,** a psychiatrist in private practice in Del Mar, CA. He is author of more than a dozen books, including *Healing Anxiety Naturally.* Perennial Currents.

Each year, millions of Americans reach for a prescription medication to curb feelings of anxiety. Unfortunately, the *benzodiazepine* tranquilizers doctors often prescribe can cause foggy thinking, memory loss and sleep disturbance...and are highly addictive.

Daily exercise and a low-fat, nutrient-dense diet help fortify the body against the effects of stress. If these measures fail to keep anxiety in check, ask your doctor about herbal remedies.

ST. JOHN'S WORT...

For individuals whose emotional state alternates between anxiety and depression, St. John's wort *(Hypericum perforatum)* is often a good choice.

This herb has proven to be just as effective as prescription antidepressants against mild to moderate depression. Since depression and anxiety often go hand in hand, the herb is widely recommended for anxiety—and for sleep disorders, too.

St. John's wort lowers levels of cortisol and enhances the activity of *gamma-aminobutyric acid* (GABA), a naturally occurring tranquilizer in the brain.

But you must be patient. The antianxiety effect can take four to six weeks to kick in.

CAUTION: Do *not* take St. John's wort within four weeks of taking a monoamine oxidase (MAO) inhibitor antidepressant, such as *phenelzine* (Nardil) or *tranylcypromine* (Parnate). This combination can trigger a dangerous rise in blood pressure, along with severe anxiety, fever, muscle tension and confusion.

Most studies of St. John's wort extract have involved dosages of 300 milligrams (mg) three times per day. At this level, side effects are mild.

St. John's wort does make the skin more sensitive to sunlight. People with fair skin should use extra sun protection, and those prone to cataracts should wear wraparound sunglasses.

VALERIAN...

Valerian is often helpful when chronic anxiety interferes with the ability to fall asleep or sleep through the night.

Like *triazolam* (Halcion) and other popular sleeping pills, valerian reduces the length of time it takes to fall asleep. Unlike these drugs, valerian produces an entirely "natural" sleep... and is nonaddictive.

The typical dosage of valerian is 900 mg taken one hour before bedtime. If you have chronic insomnia, valerian can take up to two weeks to provide relief.

SHOPPING FOR HERBS...

For optimum benefit, choose only *standardized* herbal extracts, which deliver the active ingredient in precise amounts...

• *St. John's wort:* Look for a product standardized to 0.3% *hypericin.*

• *Valerian:* Look for a product standardized to 0.8% *valerenic acid.*

CAUTION: Check with your doctor and/or pharmacist before taking any herbal remedy. Ask about potential side effects...and about any precautions that should be taken. If you are pregnant, over age 75, in frail health or taking multiple prescription drugs, take herbal remedies only under close medical supervision.

■

FLOAT FOR BETTER HEALTH

Source: **Peter Suedfeld, PhD,** professor of psychology at the University of British Columbia, Vancouver.

Taking a long walk is a great way to counteract psychological stress. But floating on your back inside a tank of warm water is even better.

Years of research and my own experience as a "floater" have convinced me that there's no better way to achieve deep relaxation. An hour of floating brings reductions in heart rate, respiration rate and muscle tension.

Floating has proven beneficial to people suffering from tension headaches and/or insomnia.

Floating also triggers an alert yet relaxed state of mind. Many floaters find that "tank time" is a terrific venue for solving difficult problems.

The typical flotation tank looks like a large plastic egg with a hatch at one end. The tank is filled with a foot of water and several hundred pounds of Epsom salts. The body is extremely buoyant in salt water.

Since the water is kept at body temperature, you're not really conscious of it. The sensation is like floating in space.

IF YOU'RE INTERESTED IN FLOTATION: Try it twice a week for two weeks. If you find the sessions helpful, "float" as often as you like.

Flotation tanks can be found in freestanding flotation facilities, fitness centers, holistic health centers and even some hospitals. A one-hour session typically runs $30 to $50.

It's possible to install a flotation tank in your home. A basic model will run about $1,500. Check your *Yellow Pages* under "flotation."

CAUTION: Avoid flotation tanks if you're claustrophobic, or if you have sores or scrapes on your skin. Pregnant women should consult a doctor before trying flotation.

■

HERBAL HEALING

HERBAL REMEDIES—
SECRETS OF GREATER EFFECTIVENESS,
SECRETS OF SAFER USE

Source: **Ethan Russo, MD,** clinical assistant professor of medicine at the University of Washington School of Medicine, Seattle. He is author of *The Handbook of Psychotropic Herbs.* Haworth Press.

People often assume that because herbs are "natural," they pose little risk. Not true.

Some herbs are too toxic for medicinal use. Even some that are generally safe can cause liver or kidney damage.

And like drugs, herbal remedies can react dangerously with certain drugs or foods.

How can you use herbal remedies for maximum safety and effectiveness? **HERE ARE SOME GUIDELINES...**

• *Avoid herbs known to be dangerous.* Given their inherent dangers, it's best to avoid chaparral, comfrey, life root, germander, coltsfoot and sassafras.

• *Don't be misled by far-fetched claims.* Federal law forbids herbal remedy manufacturers from claiming their products offer outright cures. But they often tout their products as pro-viding relief from a ludicrously wide range of ailments.

Take manufacturers' claims with a grain of salt. The best manufacturers often make no health claims for their products.

• *Seek reliable information.* The average doctor knows little about herbs. The same is true for the average druggist.

Health food store clerks may sound knowledgeable, but their information often comes from herbal remedy manufac-turers—hardly a source of unbiased information.

The most reliable source of information on herbs is *The Complete German Commission E Monographs: Therapeutic Guide to Herbal Medicines.* American Botanical Council.*

• *Work with a knowledgeable practitioner.* For referral to an herb-savvy medical doctor in your area, contact the American Botanical Council at 512-926-4900...or check out its Web site at *www.herbalgram.org.*

ALTERNATIVE: See a naturopathic physician. In addition to basic medical training, naturopaths have extensive instruc-tion in the safe use of herbs.

• *Buy only standardized formulations.* Standardized herbal extracts have been formulated to provide the active ingredient or ingredients at a specific concentration. That way, you're assured the product is both potent and safe to use.

Look for the word "standardized" or the words "German standards" on the label.

• *Follow label directions carefully.* Like drugs, herbs work best at specific dosages. Take only the recommended dosage, and be sure to take the herb with or without meals, water, etc.—as indicated.

• *Don't mix herbs and drugs.* Herbs can boost the potency of certain medications. If you're taking a prescription drug, don't begin taking any herbal extract until you've checked with a physician or naturopath.

If a doctor has prescribed a drug for you, let him/her know about any herbal remedies you are already taking. He may need to adjust the dosage.

*Your library may have this book. If not, it can be ordered from the American Botanical Council ...or via an on-line bookseller.

Common herb–drug interactions include...

• St. John's wort and *fluoxetine* (Prozac). The combination can raise brain levels of the neurotransmitter serotonin. "Serotonin syndrome" can cause delirium and other symptoms.

• Ginkgo biloba and anticoagulants. Like aspirin, *warfarin* (Coumadin) and other anticoagulants, ginkgo thins the blood. Taken along with an anticoagulant, ginkgo can cause internal bleeding.

• *Watch out for allergic reactions.* Introduce herbs one at a time. Don't add a second herb until you've taken the first for an entire week without experiencing any symptoms of an allergic reaction—rash, upset stomach, dizziness or headache.

If you experience any of these symptoms, stop taking the herb at once. Try taking it again one week later. If symptoms return, stop taking the herb for good.

CAUTION: If you become short of breath after taking an herb, call for an ambulance at once.

• *Don't take herbs during pregnancy.* Ginger, garlic and other herbs that are popular as foods are generally okay. But other herbs can cause serious problems for pregnant women.

It's also best to check with a doctor before giving any herbal remedy to a child under age 12.

■

YOU ARE WHAT YOU EAT

Source: **Neal Barnard, MD,** president of the Physicians Committee for Responsible Medicine, Washington, DC, and author of *Foods That Fight Pain.* Harmony Books.

If you experience muscle or joint pain, certain foods make excellent painkillers.

FOR MUSCLE SORENESS OR ARTHRITIC PAIN: Take one-half to one teaspoon of ginger daily—dry or fresh, cooked into recipes or in boiling water as tea. Ginger helps nausea and motion sickness, too.

ALSO FOR PAIN RELIEF: Green leafy vegetables and beans.

FOODS THAT CAN WORSEN PAIN: Dairy products...chocolate (especially bad for migraine)...eggs...citrus fruits...meat, poultry and fish...wheat.

■

GINGER FOR UPSET STOMACH...AND MORE

Source: **Stephen Fulder, PhD,** a biochemist and private research consultant in Galilee, Israel, and a former lecturer at London University. He is author of numerous books, including *The Ginger Book: The Ultimate Home Remedy.* Avery.

If you're like most Americans, the closest you get to ginger is an occasional glass of ginger ale.

But in many parts of Asia ginger is highly valued as a medicine. It's part of daily life for billions of people—as a safe, effective home remedy for a variety of ailments, including stomach upset, the common cold and poor circulation.

Powdered ginger—in the spice section at the supermarket —is potent enough. But fresh ginger is even more potent...and organic fresh ginger more potent still. **HOW TO USE GINGER...**

• *Stomach upset.* A ginger "tea" made with one-third teaspoon of powdered ginger (or one teaspoon of grated ginger) in a cup of hot water with a squeeze of lemon provides fast relief for motion sickness, nausea, vomiting or simple indigestion.

You can also buy ginger capsules or tablets at health food stores. Take two 500-milligram (mg) capsules.

Ginger calms the stomach, stopping the sensation of nausea, and speeds the digestive process.

• *Common cold.* Take two cups of ginger tea (or two 500-mg capsules) three times a day.

• *Poor circulation.* For cold hands and/or feet, take one cup of ginger tea (or a 500-mg ginger capsule) once a day, preferably in the morning. You won't see results quickly—it's more of a preventive measure than a cure.

■

PEPPERMINT FOR INTESTINAL PAIN

Source: **Larry Kincheloe, MD,** an obstetrician–gynecologist who makes extensive use of herbal medicines in his private practice in Oklahoma City.

Did you know that the familiar custom of having an after-dinner mint is rooted in herbal medicine?

KEY INGREDIENT: Peppermint oil. It facilitates digestion by soothing the stomach lining and relaxing intestinal muscles.

In addition to being a good digestive aid, peppermint oil is an effective natural remedy for *irritable bowel syndrome* (IBS). IBS is a common, stress-related disorder marked by painful spasms of the intestinal tract.

An IBS attack typically begins with nausea, vomiting and a cold, clammy feeling. Abdominal pain comes in waves.

Several prescription medications are effective at blocking the intestinal spasms, including *hyoscyamine* (Levsin). But these drugs can cause drowsiness. Peppermint oil works without causing drowsiness.

When I treat IBS patients, I typically recommend four to six cups of peppermint tea a day—which, of course, contains peppermint oil—until symptoms subside.

Peppermint tea can be made from fresh or dried peppermint leaves, which are available at health food stores and supermarkets. For each cup of hot water, use one-half ounce of fresh leaves (in small pieces) or one tablespoon of dried leaves. Steep for 10 minutes before drinking.

If you prefer store-bought peppermint tea, be sure to purchase genuine peppermint tea—made from peppermint leaves —not peppermint-flavored tea.

CAUTION: Avoid peppermint oil if you have a gastric ulcer. Pregnant women should take peppermint oil only under medical supervision.

■

RED-HOT RELIEF FOR COLD FEET AND HANDS

Source: **Andrew L. Rubman, ND,** associate professor of clinical medicine at I.W. Lane College of Integrative Medicine, Winter Park, FL. He is also medical director of the Southbury Clinic for Traditional Medicines, Southbury, CT.

You may know that a cayenne pepper extract called *capsaicin* (Capzasin) can be used topically to relieve arthritis pain. But cayenne can also be used to keep feet and hands warm in cold weather.

People whose extremities tend to be uncomfortably cold when they venture outdoors often rely upon thick insulation and/or the heat-generating chemical gel packs. But cayenne powder—one-eighth of a teaspoon sprinkled into each shoe and/or glove—acts *internally* to help the body generate heat. That's a more effective way to stay warm.

HOW IT WORKS: Water-soluble components in cayenne dilate capillaries in the skin surface, producing an immediate sensation of heat. Within 15 minutes, oil-soluble compounds reach deeper tissues, generating warmth for hours.

If you're planning to spend several hours in the cold, consider using cayenne liniment instead of cayenne powder. Liniment takes three weeks to be ready, so be sure to make a batch in advance.

WHAT TO DO: Mix one teaspoon of cayenne powder with one pint of soy oil in a bottle made of dark glass or opaque plastic. Let the contents blend for three weeks, shaking the bottle daily.

Using a dropper, rub three drops onto the soles of your feet or your hands. Wash your hands before touching your eyes.

CAUTION: Use cayenne only on unbroken skin. If irritation occurs, run cool water over the affected skin...and stop using cayenne.

Cayenne is sold in small spice bottles at grocery stores. However, it's more potent and less costly when purchased in bulk from a health food store.

Soy oil is sold in supermarkets and health food stores.

■

VITAMIN B-2 EASES MIGRAINES

Source: **Fred Sheftell, MD,** cofounder and director of The New England Center for Headache, Stamford, CT.

More than half the migraine sufferers who took 400 milligrams of vitamin B-2 daily for four months reported at least half the number of headaches they had experienced without the vitamin.

Vitamin B-2 seems to be as effective as drug treatments for migraines, with fewer side effects. Talk with your doctor before trying B-2 supplements.

■

FIVE HEALING FOODS
FOR YOUR REGULAR DIET

Source: **Jamison Starbuck, ND,** a naturopathic physician in family practice and a lecturer at the University of Montana, both in Missoula. She is past president of the American Association of Naturopathic Physicians and a contributing editor to *The Alternative Advisor: The Complete Guide to Natural Therapies and Alternative Treatments.* Time Life.

Of all the questions I get from my patients, none is more common than, "Doctor, what foods should I eat?" Here are my favorite foods. They're tasty, easy to prepare and available in grocery or health food stores. And unlike white flour products, luncheon meats, soft drinks and the other foods that many of us subsist on, these foods can help prevent—and even treat—certain illnesses.

• *Beets.* Both the red root—the part we ordinarily eat—and the green tops—the part we throw away—are full of magnesium and iron. These minerals are essential to good health.

But watch out. Like spinach, beet tops are rich in *oxalic acid.* This compound has been linked to the formation of kidney stones. Beet tops are off-limits for anyone with stones or a history of stones. The red part is safe.

Beet tops can be torn like lettuce and added to salads. They can be steamed and added to soup—or served as you would serve spinach.

You can also eat beet roots raw. Grate directly into salad …or onto a sandwich made with lettuce, onion, tuna or fresh turkey and whole grain bread.

• *Kale.* I eat this dark, leafy green veggie at least twice a week during winter and early spring. At this time of year, the body's need for vitamins and minerals rises—the result of reduced exposure to sunlight and consumption of fresh food.

Kale is a fabulous source of calcium, iron, vitamins C and A, folic acid and chlorophyll. Unlike corn, beans and tomatoes, kale can be found fresh all year long.

Kale improves circulation and helps ward off colds. The compounds that give kale its bitter flavor help improve digestion and decrease the production of mucus.

Lightly steamed kale is delicious. It tastes a bit like spinach, though more flavorful. I eat the whole leaf, but you may want to avoid the stems. They can be tough.

• *Nuts.* Brazil nuts, almonds, filberts and walnuts are packed with minerals, folic acid, vitamins B and E and beneficial oils.

I recommend buying nuts in their shells—for two reasons. First, the shell keeps nut oil from going rancid. Second, the effort required to crack each nut by hand helps ensure that you won't eat too many of these nutritious—but calorie-dense—treats.

• *Parsley.* Though best known as a garnish, parsley has much more to offer. It improves digestion, freshens the breath and curbs breast tenderness associated with premenstrual syndrome. It's also a tonic for the adrenal glands, which can become "exhausted" as a result of hard work or stress.

I like to add abundant amounts of chopped raw parsley to salads or pasta, or simply eat sprigs as a snack. Ounce for ounce, parsley contains *three times* as much vitamin C as an orange.

Women who are pregnant or nursing should have no more than a sprig of parsley per day. More than that can cause breast milk to dry up. It can even cause premature labor.

• *Sweet potatoes.* This starchy vegetable is rich in vitamin A and other carotenoids, which are necessary for healthy eyes, skin and lungs.

Bake them or combine them with onions, garlic, tomato and chickpeas to make a hearty stew.

■

THE SUPPLEMENT THAT STOPS COLD SORES

Source: **Mark A. McCune, MD,** chief of dermatology at Humana Hospital, Overland Park, KS.

People who suffer from recurrent cold sores dread the telltale itching and tingling that herald an outbreak—and with good reason.

The fluid-filled blisters, which are caused by the *herpes simplex* virus, are painful, unsightly and highly contagious.

Nuts, seeds, chocolate and certain other foods can affect the frequency and severity of cold sore outbreaks. These foods are rich in *arginine,* an amino acid that helps the herpes virus reproduce properly.

GOOD NEWS: Cold sore outbreaks can be prevented—or significantly shortened—by taking supplements of *lysine,* an amino acid found in chicken, fish and dairy products. This contention is backed up by clinical trials—and my own experience with patients.

At high dosages, lysine causes the replicating herpesvirus to make defective copies of itself. That results in a virus that's less aggressive.

For people whose cold sores recur at six- to eight-week intervals, I often recommend 3,000 milligrams (mg) of lysine daily year-round.

When outbreaks occur less frequently, it's often best to take 3,000 mg a day at the first sign of an outbreak...and to maintain that dosage until the sore crusts over.

CAUTION: Avoid lysine pills if you're pregnant or breast-feeding.

Lysine is available at pharmacies, supermarkets and health food stores.

In cases when lysine proves ineffective, I often prescribe *valacyclovir* (Valtrex). This drug should not be taken by anyone with impaired immune function.

■

6

NATURAL
SOLUTIONS

THE GREAT SECRETS OF CHINESE HEALTH...
MADE VERY EASY TO FOLLOW

Source: **Daniel Reid,** an authority on Chinese medicine, and author of several books, including *The Complete Book of Chinese Health & Healing.* Shambhala. Mr. Reid currently lives in Thailand with his wife and children.

Traditional Chinese healing practices have been in use for several thousand years, and remain the treatments of choice in China. Increasingly now, Western doctors are recognizing the value of these "alternative" approaches to health and healing.

LOW-FAT, NEAR-VEGETARIAN DIET...

Chinese medicine emphasizes a balanced diet, consisting mainly of vegetables, fruit and rice. Some animal fat—butter, meat, fish or fowl—is generally included, *but sparingly.*

Chinese medicine stresses the careful balancing of the various kinds of foods, broken down into "yin" foods, and "yang" foods.

YIN FOODS: Raw fruits and vegetables, tofu, rice, milk, yogurt, bean sprouts and raw fish.

YANG FOODS: Cooked fruits and vegetables, tomato sauce, lentils, potatoes, oats, butter and cheese, nuts, beef, lamb, chicken and cooked fish.

DIETARY SUPPLEMENTS...

Complementing a healthful diet with food extracts, enzymes and herbs has always been a main component of Chinese healing.

Westerners who convert to the Chinese diet should take the following supplements daily—vitamin C, vitamin E, vitamin B complex, beta carotene, selenium and zinc. As with any drugs, overdosage can lead to serious problems. Ask your doctor to give you the specific daily dosages of these supplements.

Also, refer to a Chinese healer or a book on Chinese medicine about food–enzyme supplements, ginseng and detoxification herbs. Overdosage of herbs, too, can be dangerous.

DIAPHRAGMATIC BREATHING...

Proper breathing is an essential part of Chinese health practices. Converts must first learn to breathe correctly at all times, breathing slowly and deeply with the diaphragm so that the abdomen expands with each inhalation and contracts with each exhalation.

Awareness of proper breathing is emphasized in *tai chi*, meditation and *chi gung* (the channeling of the breath into various parts of the body to promote the flow of health-giving chi energy).

EXERCISE...

Thirteen hundred years ago, a great Chinese physician wrote, "Flowing water never stagnates, active hinges never rust." He meant this as a metaphor for physical exercise, which keeps the spine and joints (hinges) supple, and promotes a healthy flow of the body's blood, lymph and other fluids (water) to all parts of the body.

By far the best form of exercise is traditional chi gung movements. They supplement the chi gung diaphragmatic breathing mentioned above. These slow movements are performed along with diaphragmatic breathing, while at the same time keeping a calm and quiet mind.

SEXUAL DISCIPLINE...

Traditional Chinese healing views sex as a powerful energy practice.

KEY: Control of male ejaculation and/or female orgasm.

The emphasis in Chinese medicine is on transforming sexual fluids and arousal into transcendent, healing energy—and learning to exchange this energy with your partner.

BALANCE AND HARMONY...

A fundamental element of Chinese healing is locating all forms of imbalance and disharmony in the human system, and then correcting them so that the body's healing energy (chi) can flow freely. **THIS BALANCING CAN TAKE VARIOUS FORMS, SUCH AS...**

• *Balancing yin and yang* (the basic polarity of all systems, including the human body).

• The yang diseases include fever, constipation, excessive sweating and high blood pressure. They are treated with cooling herbs and other methods that promote yin.

• The yin ailments, such as chills, diarrhea, low vitality, weakness in the limbs and aversion to cold, are treated with warming herbs and other methods that promote yang energy, while sedating yin energy.

• *Harmonizing the Five Elemental Energies—Wood, Fire, Earth, Metal and Water.* These energies represent the tangible activity of yin and yang, and encompass all the phenomena of nature.

• *Balancing the internal body with the external environment.* Eating warming yang foods, for example, when the weather is cold or damp creates such a balance.

EMPTINESS...

Eliminating clutter from all aspects of your life is a key element of Chinese health and well-being. **EXAMPLES...**

• *Adopting simplicity in diet, dress, lodgings.*

• *Learning to live with stillness and silence* (both forms of emptiness).

- *Learning the power of nonaction* and the value of "what is not."
- *Emptying the mind of mental clutter through meditation.*

SUNLIGHT...

Making sure your eyes and skin receive sufficient sunlight each day is another tenet of traditional Chinese healing. Western scientists are now advising the same approach for the millions of people who suffer winter mood disorders—since sunlight actually stimulates the pineal gland to produce important brain chemicals.

Special eye exercises can be done to help a person better absorb the beneficial rays of the sun.

However, sunbathing for merely cosmetic purposes should be avoided.

EMOTIONAL EQUILIBRIUM...

Chinese medicine identifies seven basic emotions—anger, joy, anxiety, concentration, grief, fear, fright.

As Western doctors now recognize, each emotion triggers its own set of physiological reactions.

Chinese healers believe that good health depends on keeping your emotions moderated and balanced. This is accomplished by avoiding emotional extremes, practicing nutritional therapy—on the theory that emotional problems are primarily the result of a physical problem—and by employing the correct breathing technique along with meditation.

HOLISTIC MEDICAL THERAPY...

When illness does occur, Chinese healers rely on a number of traditional treatments to help restore the flow of chi and bring the patient's energy back into healthy balance.

Instead of treating the superficial symptoms, the idea is to treat the root of the illness by addressing the underlying imbalance that's causing it.

TOOLS: Acupuncture, massage, herbs, breathing and movement exercises and carefully designed fasting programs (to purge the body of toxins).

■

NATURAL REMEDIES FOR HEADACHE PAIN

Source: **Alexander Mauskop, MD,** associate professor of clinical neurology at the State University of New York Downstate Medical Center and director of the New York Headache Center, both in New York City. He is coauthor of *The Headache Alternative: A Neurologist's Guide to Drug-Free Relief.* Dell.

Which medication works best for headache pain? **THAT DEPENDS...**

• *Migraines* are usually treated with *sumatriptan* (Imitrex), *zolmitriptan* (Zomig) or another "triptan" drug.

• *Tension headaches* are usually treated with anti-inflammatory drugs like *ibuprofen* (Motrin) or *naproxen* (Aleve).

• *Cluster headaches* are usually treated with sumatriptan or inhaled oxygen.

These treatments are reliable and safe for occasional use. But when patients start to use headache medication more than twice a week, stomach upset and other side effects become a serious concern.*

For this reason, headache sufferers should be sure to ask their doctors about trying nondrug approaches as well.

DIETARY MODIFICATION...

Chronic headaches often have their origins in food sensitivities. **TO IDENTIFY THE FOOD OR FOODS THAT UNDERLIE YOUR PAIN, TRY THIS ELIMINATION DIET...**

• *For one week, keep a list of all foods and beverages you consume.* Be sure to include seasonings.

• *For the next 30 days, avoid all foods and beverages you consumed during the 24 hours preceding each headache* you had during the week.

• *After 30 days, reintroduce suspect foods—one per meal.* Before eating the food, take your resting pulse. Twenty minutes after eating, take your pulse again.

If your pulse after eating is 10 beats or more per minute faster than your pulse before eating, you may be sensitive to the food you've just reintroduced. Avoid the food for another

*See a doctor at once if your headache is accompanied by confusion, convulsions or loss of consciousness...pain in the eye or ear...slurred speech, numbness, blurred vision or trouble walking...fever or nausea.

30 days. If you remain sensitive to this food for several months, eliminate it from your diet permanently.

NUTRITIONAL SUPPLEMENTS...

Headaches occur less frequently in individuals whose intake of certain key nutrients is adequate. **ASK YOUR DOCTOR ABOUT TAKING...**

• *Magnesium* (400 milligrams [mg] a day). This mineral has no effect on tension headaches but is moderately effective against migraines and cluster headaches.

MOST EFFECTIVE: Slow-release or chelated magnesium tablets. They're better absorbed than conventional tablets.

• *Fish oil or flaxseed oil* (15 grams [g] per day). These oils are rich in omega-3 fatty acids, which have been associated with reduced migraine frequency and severity.

• *Lecithin* (200 mg a day). This protein—sold as a powder that can be mixed into beverages—reduces the symptoms of cluster headaches.

• *Vitamin B-2* (riboflavin). Megadoses of this B vitamin—400 mg a day for two to three months—have been shown to reduce the frequency and severity of migraines.

Megadoses should be taken only under a doctor's supervision.

ACUPUNCTURE...

Acupuncture works against tension and migraine headaches. Typically, the patient undergoes sessions weekly or twice weekly for 10 weeks, followed by monthly "maintenance" sessions.

For the name of an acupuncturist in your area, contact the American Academy of Medical Acupuncture at 323-937-5514 or *www.medicalacupuncture.org.*

CAUTION: Make sure that the acupuncturist uses disposable needles.

In many cases, headaches can be prevented via acupressure, the self-help variant of acupuncture. **TRY THESE TECHNIQUES AT THE FIRST SIGN OF PAIN...**

• *Press your thumbs against the hollows between the muscles in the neck*—just below the base of the skull and in line with your ears. Hold for two minutes. Breathe deeply throughout.

• *Use your thumbs to press the upper inside corners of the eye sockets.* Hold for one minute while breathing deeply.

• *Use your right thumb to press on the top of the fleshy mound between your left thumb and index finger.* Hold for one minute while breathing deeply. Switch hands and repeat.

ENVIRONMENTAL FACTORS...

To avoid the eyestrain that triggers some headaches, be sure to have adequate lighting for the task at hand.

TRAP: Fluorescent bulbs often produce a barely perceptible flicker that can cause headaches. If there's a chance fluorescent flicker is behind your headaches, switch to incandescent bulbs.

IMPORTANT: Have a professional eye exam once a year. Straining to compensate for poor vision can cause headaches.

Mold, dust mites and fungi can trigger headaches. To eliminate these airborne irritants, install exhaust fans in your bathroom and kitchen...and a dehumidifier in your basement or any other damp area. Indoor humidity should stay between 35% and 40%.

Use scent-free hypoallergenic soap and nonaerosol sprays.

Some headaches are triggered by chronic low-level exposure to carbon monoxide (CO). Never leave a car idling in an attached garage. Consider installing a CO detector in your home.

HERBAL REMEDIES...

Feverfew can reduce the frequency as well as severity of migraines. If you'd like to try this herb, chew two fresh or freeze-dried leaves a day...or take 125 mg of dried feverfew that contains at least 0.2% *parthenolide.*

There's no evidence that herbal remedies are effective for tension or cluster headaches.

MASSAGE THERAPY...

Massage has been found to reduce the pain caused by tension and migraine headaches—but not cluster headaches.

For a referral to a massage therapist in your area, contact the American Massage Therapy Association at 877-905-2700, *www. amtamassage.org.*

BIOFEEDBACK...

By using devices that measure muscle tension and blood flow, biofeedback teaches you how to relax tense muscles... and boost blood flow to your scalp. Each technique can ease headache pain.

For adults, 10 or more 30- to 60-minute sessions may be necessary. Children typically need only five or six.

To find a biofeedback therapist in your area, send a self-addressed, stamped, business-sized envelope to the Biofeedback Certification Institute of America, 10200 W. 44th Ave., Suite 310, Wheat Ridge, Colorado 80033. Or call 303-420-2902 or visit their Web site at *www.bcia.org.*

EXERCISE...

Aerobic activity is beneficial for people who have chronic headaches. Adding a *mantra*—a word repeated over and over to focus the mind—enhances the effect.

CAUTION: Exercising during a headache tends to intensify the pain.

FOR PERSISTENT HEADACHES...

If nondrug therapies fail to work within three months, consult a headache specialist. For a listing of specialists in your area, contact the National Headache Foundation (NHF) at 888-NHF-5552 or *www.headaches.org*...or send a self-addressed, stamped, business-sized envelope to the NHF at 820 N. Orleans, Suite 217, Chicago 60610.

STOP MUSCLE PAIN IN 90 SECONDS

Source: **Dale Anderson, MD,** adjunct assistant professor at the University of Minnesota Medical School, Minneapolis. He is author of *Muscle Pain Relief in 90 Seconds.* John Wiley & Sons.

Using a simple "fold-and-hold" technique, it's possible to stop most muscular aches in less time than it takes to make a doctor's appointment.

Fold-and-hold involves no drugs, dietary supplements or special instruments—just four simple steps...

1. *Find the tender spot.*

2. *Move your body into a position that minimizes the pain.* This usually involves "folding" one part of the body over another to reduce tension on the underlying muscle.

3. *Hold the folded position for 90 seconds.* Then slowly return to the original position.

4. *Gently stretch in the opposite direction.*

Fold-and-hold is especially useful for...

• ***Bunions.*** Twist the big toe under the foot and push toward the center of the foot. Do this yourself—or with the help of another person. Hold and release.

• ***Heel spurs*** (plantar fasciitis). Fold the bottom of your foot by pushing the heel and toes together. Although it's easier to get someone to do this for you as you lie on your stomach, you can do it yourself by pushing the top of your foot against the seat of a chair. Hold and release.

If fold-and-hold doesn't work after three tries, see a doctor. If fold-and-hold worsens your pain, stop immediately.

■

AROMATHERAPY—ESSENTIAL OILS TO SOOTHE YOUR SOUL AND HEAL YOUR BODY

Source: **Kurt Schnaubelt, PhD,** scientific director of the Pacific Institute of Aromatherapy, San Rafael, CA. He is author of *Advanced Aromatherapy—The Science of Essential Oil Therapy* (Inner Traditions) and *Medical Aromatherapy* (Frog Ltd.).

Aromatherapy involves the use of *essential oils*—the distilled aromatic essence of various plants—which can be either inhaled or applied to the skin.

Essential oils may also be taken internally, but this can be *risky,* and should be done only under the supervision of a trained aromatherapist.

GETTING STARTED...

While certain oils may be used to treat specific illnesses, many essential oils help promote general health and relaxation as well. Their aromatic molecules act as tonics to the nervous system, helping to restore its equilibrium.

Aromatherapy is especially effective for treating stress-related disorders and other nervous system or hormonal imbalances.

Some oils have also been shown to boost immune system function…and/or to reduce inflammation.

Because everyone responds a bit differently to various essential oils, I recommend taking a playful approach to aromatherapy, experimenting freely with up to 10 different scents to begin with.

CAUTION: To be sure you're not allergic to any of the essential oils listed below, test each one before using it. Apply a drop to the skin on the inside of your elbow, then wait for 24 hours. If no redness or swelling appears, the oil is generally safe for you to use.

HOW TO USE ESSENTIAL OILS...

For beginners at aromatherapy, there are several recommended ways to use essential oils.

Essential oils can be inhaled by…

• *Putting a drop or two on your pillow before going to sleep.*

• *Putting a drop or two on a small piece of cotton or paper towel,* then placing the cotton or paper towel directly into your nostril.

• *Using an electronic diffuser.* The diffuser sends minuscule oil droplets into the air.

Essential oils can also be applied to the skin—where they then quickly work their way into the tissues below. **THIS CAN BE DONE BY…**

• *Adding five to 10 drops to your bath water.*

• *Pausing in the middle of a shower to rub a small handful* (five to 10 drops) of essential oil over your body.

• *Mixing essential oils with a massage oil "base"*—adding 10 drops of essential oil for each ounce of massage oil.

I recommend using either sesame oil or hazelnut oil as bases, since both are light oils with a mild, pleasant fragrance. Almond, avocado and sunflower oil make good bases as well.

TREATING SPECIFIC PROBLEMS...

There are dozens of essential oils in wide use today, each with their own healing properties.

Here are some of the most common health applications of aromatherapy and the essential oils best suited for each use...

• *General relaxation.* I recommend lavender, geranium or clary sage oil. These oils can either be dispersed into the air with a diffuser, added to bath water or rubbed over the body via massage oil.

Inhaling mandarin oil is also effective for reducing anxiety.

• *Skin problems.* Lavender oil applied directly into the skin is often an effective treatment for skin irritations as long as the skin is not broken, and it is good for general skin health as well.

Tea tree oil, which has antibacterial properties, is also effective at treating skin problems—especially acne, herpes and infections of the mouth and gums.

• *Insomnia or restlessness.* Before going to bed, place a few drops of orange or mandarin oil directly on your pillow (it may stain) or on a piece of cotton by your bedside. Both of these oils are deeply relaxing, and have an extremely pleasant fragrance.

• *Upper-respiratory infections.* If someone in your house has a bad cold or flu, the airborne microorganisms that cause these illnesses can be sharply reduced by using a diffuser to spread droplets of eucalyptus or lavender oil (or a mixture of the two) into the air. This will help prevent the sickness from spreading to other family members.

The person with the cold or flu may speed his/her healing process by standing directly over the diffuser and inhaling these oil droplets.

Another option is ravensare oil, which is good for treating flu symptoms and also has an emotionally uplifting effect.

• *Boost immune system function.* For general health, bay laurel is one of the most invigorating of all essential oils.

You can strengthen your immune system by inhaling the oil or applying it topically in a massage oil base, especially to the skin above the lymph glands, since it's especially good for the lymphatic system.

This approach is particularly recommended to help alleviate the discomfort of swollen lymph nodes.

• *Sprains, aches, cuts and other minor injuries.* Applying a mixture of everlasting oil and massage oil onto the affected area will help reduce swelling and pain, and speed healing.

This oil has a unique blend of anti-inflammatory and analgesic properties. If applied quickly to a bruise, it prevents hemorrhaging as well. Everlasting oil is also effective in reducing the joint pain associated with rheumatoid arthritis.

• *Gastrointestinal disturbances.* Minor digestive problems can often be eased by ingesting rosemary or tarragon oil.

• *Enhance sensuality and sexuality.* Diffuse oil of lavender or jasmine (an especially potent sensual enhancer) in the room— or apply a few drops to your pillows and sheets. You can also employ one or both oils in a massage oil base.

■

ELECTROSTATIC MASSAGE

Source: **Milton Hammerly, MD,** medical director, integrative medicine, Catholic Health Initiatives, Denver.

Did you know that *static electricity* is an effective remedy for headaches, arthritis and other common sources of pain?

Physicians have long recognized that the human body is pulsing with minute electrical currents. "Normalizing" this disrupted flow of electricity promotes healing. In fact, doctors have been using low-voltage electrical currents to mend broken bones.

A similar effect can be obtained using static electricity. Sweeping a charged object across a painful or injured region of the body attracts a flow of healing electric current to the area.

Doing so also speeds the circulation of fluid away from the area, thereby reducing swelling.

To do "electrostatic massage" (EM), you'll need a one-foot section of polyvinyl chloride (PVC) pipe, 1.5 inches in diameter ...plus an ordinary painter's mitt. These items are available at hardware stores.

WHAT TO DO: Rub the pipe vigorously with the mitt for one minute, then slowly sweep the pipe over the painful area. Move in a head-to-toe direction—one-quarter to one-half inch away from the skin.

I usually recommend two 15-minute electrostatic massage sessions each day for as long as pain persists.

■

7

VERY PERSONAL

SEXUAL AROMATHERAPY

Source: **Alan R. Hirsch, MD,** neurological director of the Smell & Taste Treatment and Research Foundation, 845 N. Michigan Ave., Suite 990W, Chicago 60611, *www.smellandtaste.org.* He is author of *Scentsational Sex: The Secret to Using Aroma for Arousal.* HarperCollins.

The seductive images in perfume ads would have us believe that the costliest fragrances are the most erotic.

Pleasant scents *do* enhance sexual pleasure. That's been proven again and again. But the scents that pack the most powerful aphrodisiac punch might surprise you.

My research has shown that the aromas of certain foods—including some you would never suspect—are far more arousing than even the costliest perfume.

In fact, our research showed that men's cologne was a strong *turnoff* for many women.

SCENTS AROUSING TO MEN: Pumpkin pie combined with lavender...cinnamon buns...and black licorice combined with doughnuts.

If you'd like to try these aromas on your partner, keep pie, buns or doughnuts in a warm oven. That will spread the aromas.

Lavender is available as a candle, in room-freshening sprays or as essential oil. What about licorice? Offer your partner some licorice candy.

SCENTS AROUSING TO WOMEN: Good 'n Plenty candy combined with cucumber...baby powder...and pumpkin pie linked with lavender.

To try these aromas on your partner, you might offer her some Good 'n Plenty candy after dinner. Peel and slice the cucumber, then eat it...or rub it on your bodies. Sprinkle baby powder on your bodies or sheets.

The food–sex link makes perfect sense in evolutionary terms. Only when food was plentiful did our distant ancestors have the opportunity to procreate.

It's also possible that these food aromas simply elicit a sense of nostalgia that makes people feel comfortable—and therefore sexy.

■

VIAGRA ALTERNATIVES

Source: **Adriane Fugh-Berman, MD,** medical adviser, National Women's Health Network, Washington, DC, and author of *Alternative Medicine: What Works.* Lippincott, Williams & Wilkins.

Extracts of ginkgo leaves or ginseng root are natural alternatives to Viagra for treating impotence. They are available at drugstores and health food stores. Consult your physician before trying either remedy. **THESE ARE THE DOSAGES THAT I WOULD DISCUSS...**

GINKGO: 40 milligrams (mg) extract, three times a day. Don't use it if you take aspirin or blood thinners.

GINSENG: 100 mg to 200 mg extract daily. Men using ginseng should have their blood pressure monitored regularly. Don't use it if you drink caffeinated beverages regularly or take other stimulants.

And be patient—it may take several months to see results.

■

HERBAL HELP FOR PMS

Source: The late **Varro E. Tyler, PhD,** former professor emeritus of pharma-cognosy at Purdue University, West Lafayette, IN. He is author of *Tyler's Herbs of Choice: The Therapeutic Use of Phytomedicinals.* Haworth Press.

Folklore has it that monks used the peppery fruit of the chasteberry bush *(Vitex agnus-castus)* to suppress their sexual desires.

Today chasteberry is used by women as a natural remedy for premenstrual syndrome (PMS) and other ailments caused by hormone imbalances.

Support for the use of chasteberry comes from a distinguished panel of German scientists, who completed a lengthy review of research on herbal remedies.

The panel recommended chasteberry for bloating, headache, depression and other symptoms of PMS...for menopausal hot flashes...and for painful breasts.

Chasteberry acts on the pituitary gland, a pea-sized gland located at the base of the brain. In turn, the pituitary gland signals the ovaries to restore a normal balance of the hormones estrogen and progesterone.

If you'd like to try chasteberry, consult your doctor to be sure that your symptoms stem from a hormone imbalance.

For PMS, chasteberry generally should be taken from the very onset of symptoms until the beginning of the menstrual period.

For other problems, chasteberry can be taken continuously for up to six months.

The usual dose is 20 milligrams (mg) per day. To avoid side effects—typically, mild gastrointestinal problems such as nausea—take chasteberry with meals.

CAUTION: Chasteberry should be avoided by women who are pregnant or on hormone therapy.

Chasteberry is available in health food stores as a liquid extract or in capsule form.

■

ALTERNATIVES TO HORMONE THERAPY

Source: **Jamison Starbuck, ND,** a naturopathic physician in family practice and a lecturer at the University of Montana, both in Missoula. She is past president of the American Association of Naturopathic Physicians and a contributing editor to *The Alternative Advisor: The Complete Guide to Natural Therapies and Alternative Treatments.* Time Life.

Thousands of women are now deciding against hormone-replacement therapy (HRT), and I can't say I blame them. For decades, HRT was the treatment of choice for menopausal women. It helps to curb menopausal symptoms—hot flashes, vaginal dryness, insomnia and mood swings. HRT also seems to reduce the risk for osteoporosis.

But HRT has important drawbacks. Earlier claims that it lowers the risk of heart disease and Alzheimer's disease have not been proven by recent studies. And, one recent study found that in women with existing heart trouble, HRT actually increases the likelihood of dangerous blood clots. In addition, estrogen only prevents the loss of bone tissue, while *isoflavones*—a natural alternative to estrogen found in soy foods—actually promote the growth of new bone tissue. Perhaps most disturbing, HRT appears to raise the risk for breast cancer.

Consider these suggestions...

• *Take control of your situation.* Ask your doctor for a comprehensive physical exam, and review your personal and family health history. HRT is an especially bad idea for women with a strong family history of breast cancer. Consider your risk for heart disease and osteoporosis, and make sure you're doing all you can to avoid these illnesses. If you're not eating well and getting regular exercise, get started. Aerobic exercise in particular—20 minutes, four times a week—has been shown to be effective against hot flashes and menopausal depression.

• *Eat soy foods every day.* Hot flashes can be reduced, and perhaps even eliminated, by drinking 16 ounces of soy milk each day...or eating soy powder containing 50 milligrams (mg) of isoflavones each day. Soy powder can be blended with yogurt, fruit and nuts for a breakfast drink...or sprinkled on hot cereal.

• *Consider herbal remedies.* When menopausal patients come to me complaining about mood swings, depression or insomnia,

I often recommend *black cohosh* (Cimicifuga racemosa). This herb is also great for hot flashes. The typical dosage is one-quarter teaspoon of tincture twice a day.

If anxiety and heart palpitations are a problem, I often recommend two to four cups per day of an herbal tea made from one part each of linden leaves, hawthorn flowers, passion flower and chamomile. Combine all the herbs in a jar. Steep one tablespoon of the herb mixture in eight ounces of boiling water for at least five minutes, then strain before drinking.

• *Do some additional reading.* I particularly like *The Herbal Menopause Book* (Crossing Press), by Amanda McQuade Crawford...and I recommend *Natural Woman, Natural Menopause* (HarperCollins), by Marcus Laux, ND, and Christine Conrad.

■

SEX IS VERY GOOD FOR YOUR HEALTH

Source: **Beverly Whipple, PhD, RN,** certified sex educator, counselor, researcher and professor emerita at Rutgers University–Newark. She is coauthor of the international best-seller *The G-Spot and Other Recent Discoveries About Human Sexuality.* Dell. She was a consultant for the report *The Health Benefits of Sexual Expression* for Planned Parenthood Federation of America, Inc.

A recent review of dozens of studies shows that sexual expression is good for the heart...the immune system...the reproductive system...and for controlling pain, stress and depression. It may even extend your life. It seems that sex triggers the release of many powerful chemicals in the body.

BENEFITS...

• *Longevity.* A Welsh study of more than 900 men ages 45 to 59 showed that those who averaged two or more orgasms per week had half the risk of dying during the 10-year period of the study, compared with those who had orgasms less than once a month. In addition to the Welsh study, a study of 252 men and women in North Carolina showed that frequency of sexual intercourse was a significant predictor of longevity for men.

In a Swedish study of 392 older men and women, married men who stopped having sex before the age of 70 were more likely to die by age 75 than married men who continued to be sexually active (for women, there was no association between sexual intercourse and mortality).

• *Heart disease.* In the Welsh study, men who had orgasms less than once a month had twice the rate of fatal heart attacks, compared with men who had orgasms two or more times a week.

POSSIBLE EXPLANATION: The hormone DHEA is released during orgasms. Research on middle-aged men suggests that the lower the level of DHEA in the blood, the higher the risk of heart disease.

• *Breast cancer.* In a French study of 146 women ages 25 to 45 who had never had children, those who had sexual intercourse less than once a month had a higher risk of breast cancer than those who had sex more often.

POSSIBLE EXPLANATION: Sexual arousal and orgasm leads to increased levels of the sex hormone *oxytocin,* which may help prevent breast cancer.

• *Immunity.* Two psychology professors at Wilkes University in Pennsylvania measured levels of *immunoglobulin A* (IgA) in 112 subjects. This immune factor is essential in defeating viruses. Subjects who had sexual intercourse once or twice a week had IgA levels that were 30% higher than those who didn't have sex.

• *Pain.* Many reports in the medical literature show that sex relieves pain, including back pain, menstrual cramps, arthritis and migraine. In one study, stimulation in female lab rats caused the pelvic nerve to release the *polypeptide vasoactive intestinal peptide* (VIP). When injected into animals, VIP has a pain-blocking power stronger than morphine.

• *Insomnia.* A psychologist who surveyed 1,866 US women found that 32% had masturbated in the past three months to help get to sleep. The hormones released may act as a natural sedative.

• *Emotional health.* Studies show that sexual satisfaction is a strong predictor of higher quality of life.

EXAMPLES: A Canadian study of 75 men between the ages of 18 and 27 showed that men who were not sexually active had the highest risk of depression. And, in an American study, women who masturbate reported a higher level of self-esteem than women who don't.

Studies also show that sexual activity and orgasm reduce stress, which may be related to the release of oxytocin.

■